You Are Enough:

A Manifesto for the Overworked and Overwhelmed

You Are Enough:

A Manifesto for the Overworked and Overwhelmed

ISLIN MUNISTERI

With foreword by Stephanie Frey

ISBN 978-0-692-69969-0

Islin Ventures LLC
11018 Kaskanak Drive
Eagle River, AK 99577
www.islinmunisteri.com

Printed in the United States of America

First Printing, 2016

Library of Congress Control Number: 2016907237

Cover Design: Ana Grigoriu, https://www.books-design.com

Editing: Paper Raven Books, http://paperravenbooks.com

This book is dedicated to Nancy and Mel, because you believed in my ability to write before anyone else. Thank you.

CONTENTS

FOREWORD

"You are enough." Three simple words that hold great significance. In my professional work over the years as a licensed therapist, I've had the privilege to walk alongside hundreds of people working out this belief in their lives. In terms of one's self concept, a person's belief about their own lovability and significance shapes who they are, and has profound implications for how they choose to live their life.

Often times, a person develops core beliefs or ways of seeing and perceiving themselves through early life experiences. Usually, these experiences occur or are framed within one's family of origin. The family is the predominant socializing agent of life during our early years and what happens during these formative years is significant. Just as important are perceptions about the world, others, and ourselves that we develop as a result of our experiences. From these experiences, we develop core beliefs that can be negative, such as "I am unlovable," "I am helpless," and "I am not enough," or positive, such as "I am lovable," "I can trust others," and "I am enough."

Unfortunately, our family experiences and our perceptions are not always positive, healthy, or constructive. These beliefs often develop unconsciously and exist for years before they rear their ugly heads.

For many people, it isn't until a time of major transition

or crisis that they become aware of some of the underlying beliefs that have guided and shaped their identity.

Once aware, it is staggering to observe how deeply rooted these beliefs are and how they have influenced countless decisions. For some, the belief that they are unlovable prevents relationships, keeps them from taking risks, or leads to addiction, isolation, depression, confusion, and the list goes on and on. Of course, these feelings influence daily decisions. What would happen if their belief were that they "were lovable" or they "were enough?" In turn, it would lead to more positive feelings, choices, decisions, and behaviors. Hopefully you're beginning to see that one's beliefs have significant ramifications for their entire life.

In "You Are Enough," Islin Munisteri gives an honest, authentic, and vulnerable response to what happens when a person believes they are not enough. She bravely dives into the depths of her early childhood experiences and explores how they have shaped her sense of self. Islin challenges the reader to examine why they do what they do and if it is truly working in their life. In this day and age, we need authentic voices that are willing to be honest, vulnerable, and encouraging. Islin encourages readers, through her own life journey, while giving practical insights to guide a person through the process of accepting the truth of the following three words when they hear them: "You Are Enough."

Stephanie Frey, LPC, LMFT
April 2016
Houston, Texas
USA

PREFACE

October 2014 was the second time I thought of taking my own life.

December 2010 was the first.

During both months I had to take short-term disability leave from work to take care of "personal business at home." I called it postpartum depression, once the breastfeeding stopped, and the happy oxytocin left my bloodstream. But there was a lot more at play. I was stressed-out and angry, turning into a heartless bitch who didn't blink twice at displacing more senior engineers to get the work and the glory. I felt guilty. I felt guilty picking up the kids at 6:30 pm, getting home at 7:00 pm, and putting them to bed an hour or an hour and a half later. It couldn't go on.

The traffic on I-10 was getting to be unbearable in Houston.

Worst of all, I had false beliefs about what I had to be—perfect. A perfect mom and perfect engineer and perfect wife and perfect volunteer. Despite winning multiple awards for my work, I was never satisfied with who I was. They just made me feel more ashamed of myself.

I would show them to my mom—yes I still needed approval from my mom at 25 years of age—and she shrugged them off. I was Young Engineer of the Year in SWE Houston! I was an SWE Nominee for Engineer's Week, a national award! But no, she simply shrugged off what I had shown her, and it broke my heart. Like everything else negative, I internalized it deep, and ruminated until I was suicidal.

I questioned my validity as a family female engineer in the oilfield. Sometimes I would believe the rhetoric that they only chose me as a diversity candidate; even though I had volunteering experience, had gotten a fairly good GPA, and a bevy of scholarships during my senior year, as well as all through college.

And in December 2010, something snapped. I had to make a production profile in less than 24 hours and there was 200 million dollars on the line. I was a nervous wreck, running on five hours of sleep from taking care of my one-year-old. I couldn't take the pressure. My technical mentor sneered at me, and I cracked.

After two weeks of group therapy and trial by being asked "are you feeling suicidal on this anti-depressant?" by a psychiatrist, and the holidays, I went back to work on a nasty flatline; as flat as the lifeless landscape in Houston, where my mood was somewhere between ground level and six-feet-under. But at least I wasn't suicidal.

Right?

But in October 2014, things got worse. I had another "break" from work on short-term disability, and this time I was somewhere between ideation and attempted suicide. I remember walking up the cold cement stairs in the North garage on the campus, one at a time, until I broke free to the roof. There were dozens of pigeons huddled near a lamp. They were so free. They could fly where they wanted to go. They were not trapped to the ground. For a few moments each day, they could dive and swoop and simply be themselves—be birds.

I remember looking down from the top of the garage, and taking a deep breath, enjoy that feeling of flight.

My thoughts became incredibly clear. It was time to jump.

I could see the target pattern enumerated by the clay tiles below. Gosh, it would be so embarrassing if I didn't land in the dead center of the tile pattern, I thought. I start laughing like a banshee. Here I was at life's end, and I still wanted to end it perfectly.

My laughter startled the pigeons. Their feathered bodies shimmered against the sunset as they took off in flight, the whole two dozen of them, until they found another spot on the parking garage, this time near the furthest corner away from me. They too had to return to the ground. In that moment, their strong midnight shadow contrasting against the striking orange sunset told me to step back from the edge. Life, perhaps, was too beautiful to end on target. It was these imperfect moments of beauty that reminded me I still had a life outside of work. What about my kids and my family? What about my friends? What about my colleagues? What about my people? I started the long walk back down the cement stairs. I noticed that each floor of the parking garage was enumerated with a bright color. Purple Eight. Yellow Seven. Green Six. Orange Five. Green Four. Purple Three. Orange Two. Yellow One.

The simple colors and numbers reminded me of my children. I hurried to my car in the other garage, five minutes away by foot. I still needed to pick the kids up from day care. And it was my turn today. How horrible it would have been for my husband to find out about my death from a late day care call.

CHAPTER 1. YOU ARE MORE THAN PERFECT ALREADY.

"[B]y cramming a child's life full of activities, with little time for reflection, with no quiet time for a relaxed parent-child supper, this mom is sending an unintended message: what you do is more important than who you are.

—Dr. Leonard Sax, *The Collapse of Parenting*

Damn it, stop trying so hard. Who the hell are you trying to impress anyway? Why are you doing what you are doing? Is it to please your parents and your supervisor, or do you want to do it just for the sake of doing it, even if you were never paid again to do it?

Would you still be a whole person if you lost your job tomorrow? Your partner? Your family? Could you rebuild?

Or is it something worse in some cases? Perhaps it is intrinsic motivation gone extreme. This goes beyond impressing your boss and your family. Are you performing at a level beyond what you can sustainably support with your current energy levels? Have you gone striving to the point of perfection to fulfill an intrinsic need for self-worth and love and validation of your existence?

The point of you being more than perfect comes down the fact that perfect is static. It doesn't move; it's not changing; it has run out of entropy and

and the system is in equilibrium.

Perfect means death. Perfect means the height of whatever you're doing, which means it is all downhill from there. And that's not the case at all.

You are alive. You are not dead, which means you are not perfect.

But don't go commit suicide to prove that you are perfect. That defeats the purpose of life and of being alive.

I also know that this is an imperfect proof. This is not geometry. This is not mathematics.

But really, for all intents and purposes, you are not perfect.

And that's okay.

This took me 27 years to learn, and I think I'm still relearning this lesson every two months or so. When everything is going so well, and I can sit back in my office and I think I can just relax, something will go wrong. The kids and I come down with the flu. The dog needs to go the groomers. My husband is working 14-hour days at the office and forgets to tell me. I have a Tuesday night class that I forget to tell him about. Our au pair has suddenly worked over her hours for the day. A big meeting is coming up that I haven't adequately prepared for, or given enough of shit about to adequately prepare for. My boss and I have different goals. Everything that was on autopilot needs to have new code written because autopilot isn't working anymore.

Before, my lizard brain would take over and I would be

frozen in flight or fight mode. Every action, event or, thought, no matter how small or insignificant, would be an emergency, an earthquake that could level San Francisco. The anxiety would come and break me down like a tsunami levelling small archipelagos after the earthquake.

Now, take a deep breath, Brene Brown-style. Inhale for a count of four beats. Hold the air in your belly for a count of four beats. Exhale and push the air out of your diaphragm for four beats. Hold for four beats. Then inhale again. Feel the air go into your diaphragm and lungs. Exhale. Feel the air empty from your lungs and then your stomach.

It will be all right. You are not entitled to a perfect day, every day. Or even ever. Just be grateful for those days where everything runs smoothly and you're not powered by some traffic-induced flight-fight-freeze adrenaline rush mixed with the stress of the ticking clock telling you you're 15 minutes late to the dentist appointment—and you're still 10 minutes away.

No, you are not entitled to perfection. You are not entitled to a perfect wedding, a perfect mate, a perfect mood, a perfect set of children, a perfect boss, the perfect equation to solve life's problems, the perfect sunset, the perfect place in life, the perfectly healthy life, the perfectly healthy lifestyle, the perfect professor, the perfect advisor, the perfect resume builder, the perfect interviewer, the prefect friend, the perfect IQ, the perfect EQ, the perfect StrengthsFinder™, the perfect gymnast-ballerina-800-on-the-SAT-math-section-in-seventh-grade-child, the perfect house in the perfect neighborhood, the perfect fill-in-the-blank that you so desperately pine for.

Get over it.

This is life.
This is entropy.
This is chaos.
You are more than perfect.
You are imperfect.

One-Minute Chapter Summary

You are perfect as you are—stop trying to strive beyond your sustainable energy levels to summit the next mountain or get the next award. Some questions to ponder: who are you trying to prove yourself to anyway? Why are you pushing yourself so hard?

Make a choice now, and repeat it aloud. Whispering counts.

- I am not perfect, and I accept that fact. I am the way I am, and I choose to respect the energy level that I have and stop fighting with myself to be that "perfect" woman, mom, employee, volunteer, and all the other roles I play in my life. I accept myself the way I am, blemishes and all.
- I am perfect and will continue to strive and prove myself to exhaustion, burnout, depression, and anxiety so that I can get to the pinnacle of whatever it is that I am chasing.

Head to http://bit.ly/youareenoughquiz_to put in your answers, so that you can have a list of your affirmations and one-minute summaries to take with you after you finish reading the book.

CHAPTER 2. GET OFF THE TREADMILL.

"People may spend their whole lives climbing the ladder of success only to find, once they reach the top, that the ladder is leaning against the wrong wall."
—Thomas Merton

You know which one I'm talking about—the Hedonist Treadmill. The one that whispers in your ear, "After I get this promotion, then I'll stop working 60-hour workweeks." Or perhaps, "After I fix my kid one more organic chicken-avocado sandwich to show up Mrs. Jones over there, then I can settle back down and pack peanut butter and jelly sandwiches again."

It's a fun, destructive cycle. It keeps us in places that are unhealthy. At least it was unhealthy for me at that time to stay in corporate America. But I kept on saying to myself, "One more rotation, let's see where they put me this time."

But that's the problem with the treadmill. No matter what you do to improve your happiness level, it settles back to the same place as before you got your promotion. You just keep on jogging on it until it jogs on you. Or you get run off. You don't have a stop button or a safety button or a pause button. The Treadmill of Endless Desires never stops.

It continued this way until I finally woke up one day thinking, "I can't live like this anymore."

Something had to give. We had to move to somewhere slower. I had to have a slower job, where I wasn't firefighting every day with upper management looking over my shoulder.

I felt that something was definitely repressed. There were a lot of Pandora's boxes, and it was definitely not Hope that I saw at the bottom when all the hells of the world finally disappeared. I didn't feel whole.

A particularly kind human resource manager said to me, "You have to bring your whole self to work, honey."

She was right. I was definitely bringing a particular subset of Islin to work—the hypercompetitive, angry, I will eat you alive, I will get this done faster, never content, always hungry, un-human Islin to the office.

I had forgotten about the other, softer, gentler parts of me, because I thought it was a weakness to reveal them. These loom-weaving, ballet-dancing, yogifying parts of me didn't get the job done in the office. And so I left them on a back shelf somewhere in my four-cube pod.

But not bringing my whole self to work was detrimental to my mental and emotional health. I was fighting with myself all the time. Was I good enough? Was the engineering product I spat out good enough? Was I being a good mom? Was I being a good human being? Did I deserve to exist? The parts of me I left lying on a bookshelf longed to be integrated with the whole—even if it was competitive, ambitious, and at times angry.

Yes, I was extremely angry. And anger turned inwards becomes depression. And long-term depression easily

leads to addiction.
That's what happens when you stay on the Treadmill too long. You become addicted to the next thing, the next promotion, the next award, the next…
Until something wakes you up.
For me, that was major depression. But it took me two wake up calls before I was receptive enough to hear it.
For some people, they hear it loud and clear the first time with a health scare, or something more permanent.
It may be Stage 4 cancer. It may be not having a boyfriend or realizing that you wanted to have children, but it's almost too late.
Whatever it is that wakes you up, get off the treadmill.
It's not good for your long-term health, mental, physical, or spiritual.
Now, you may get a little beat up by getting off.
Your friends may hate you for it—you'll make them feel bad for staying on.
You'll probably need to find a different group of friends to help you stay off.
I'm not suggesting that you stop trying, that you stop living and evolving and growing.
I'm only advocating for a sense of balance.
I'm suggesting that you know when enough is enough.
I'm saying that you know that you are enough.
Right here.
Right now.
You are enough.

One-Minute Chapter Summary

Despite chasing the next promotion or the next award, once you achieve it, sometimes it feels so—empty. Are you caught on the Hedonist Treadmill? Once you get what you've been wishing for, your mood often settles back to where it was before obtaining your wish.

Make a choice now:

- I choose to get off the Hedonist Treadmill and understand why I feel the way I do, knowing that no promotions or awards will increase my inherent level of happiness.
- I choose to stay on the Hedonist Treadmill and proceed without self-awareness into my motivations. I will continue to work at my current pace until I have a major health wake up call.

Head to http://bit.ly/youareenoughquiz to put in your answers, so that you can have a list of your affirmations and one-minute summaries to take with you after you finish reading the book.

CHAPTER 3. TREAT YOURSELF WITH SELF-COMPASSION.

"You can search throughout the entire universe for someone who is more deserving of your love and affection than you are yourself, and that person is not to be found anywhere. You, yourself, as much as anybody in the entire universe, deserve your love and affection."
—Gautama Buddha

Sometimes I really hate self-compassion. Yes, I said it! It is so difficult to explain, because I don't fully understand it myself. But I know it's about giving yourself the permission to find yourself in the 30-foot seas of life. It's about believing in and becoming yourself. It is about that magical thing that makes all things possible.

Self-compassion is one of the fewest applied salves in the Western world. We give our friends, our causes, our kids, our pets, our significant other, our slacker employee, and just about everything in the universe more compassion than we give ourselves. We are so hard on ourselves. Pursuing perfection in a project or trying to get to the next promotion or whatever it is that we are doing is never quite good enough. I didn't put the oil away in the pantry in the right spot. That means the cookies won't turn out well because they weren't perfect. Everything wasn't perfect at our first try, so we failed. Luckily, life is not an all or nothing venture. Life exists in between the awards and the ego-boosts and everything that goes badly, or what we interpret as going badly. It's okay.

In fact, it's all okay. Nothing is horrible, but we can label things as horrible. Sometimes you just have to accept it as it is, and give yourself the grace. So stop yelling inside your mind that you're a bad mom if you yelled at your kids for a minor infraction. Give yourself the grace. Give yourself that space to absorb all the beauty and ugliness of human life. You feel like you are not good enough to do what you are doing? Find a way to reframe it through self-compassion. Give yourself the grace to say that it is all right, to say that it is okay to feel that way, and find a way to use that to fuel you, instead of making you feel worse, like you want to hide under the covers all day.

It is okay.

Give yourself grace, especially in the worst of moments. Don't make your worst moment worse by not giving yourself the grace to revel and be grateful that you can actually feel these emotions.

Self-compassion is incredibly difficult. But it's worth it. It's what makes learning and change possible. Self-compassion gives you the space to challenge the negative voices and the negative scripts your parents did not intentionally mean to give you. It's that magical step that makes leaps possible. Sometimes, you just have to believe that are worthy of giving yourself self-compassion. You are worthy of going beyond the negative beliefs in your mind. You are worthy of giving yourself the spaces to challenge the beliefs that you had. There was a time in my life where I would berate myself like never before for calculating something incorrectly at work. The significance of this mistake was not small; but I didn't give myself the compassion to get through it, acknowledge the mistake, and move on. I was stuck in the strange world of constantly berating myself, not feeling good enough—a vicious spiral downward.

But now I've learned that when I let the mistake go, allow myself to learn the lesson, and don't beat myself up, my productivity actually increases. I'm no longer so uptight about the outcome. I'm relaxed, and just enjoy the fact that I've actually arrived somewhere—who cares if it was the wrong conclusion initially? This mindset gives me the space to iterate, to learn again, and to fail in a different way.

Self-compassion helps you to get out of the self-destructive, self-critical hell that you put yourself through. Give yourself the kindness to say, "It's okay. I'm only human."

For any naysayers out there, would you be compassionate towards the engineer who made a mistake but caught it, or would you send her over to her manager and ask that she be removed from her job? Or would you say, "She won't do it again. Let's give her a chance. She's a pretty good person by and large, and we can't let this one mistake define her whole career?"

Or when teaching your five-year-old daughter how to read, would you send her to time out if she didn't know the word "the," even though you've gone through it half a dozen times with her? No, I hope not.

But hell, shit happens. Maybe you did make some mistakes. But how are you going to react next time or, better yet, not react at all and give yourself the gift of having self-compassion, and then act in a more thoughtful manner?

I'm not saying that you should give yourself infinite chances. I am saying that if you want to be successful, you need to be kind enough to yourself that when you fail, you tell yourself, "It's okay. I'm a big girl." Dust yourself off. Be patient with yourself.

Some people think being kind and compassionate to yourself is taboo.

Don't let it be.

Practice self-compassion.

Accept your mistakes.

They might be blessings in disguise.

Among the people who lived close to the border, there was a man who led a righteous life. Without reason, his horse escaped, and fled into barbarian territory. Everyone pitied him, but the old man said: "What makes you think this is not a good thing?"
Several months later, his horse returned, accompanied by a superb barbarian stallion. Everyone congratulated him. But the old man said: "What makes you think this is cannot be a bad thing?"
The family was richer from a good horse, his son enjoyed riding it. He fell and broke his hip. Everyone pitied him, but the old man said: "What makes you think this is not a good thing!"
One year later, a large party of barbarians entered the border. All the valid men drew their bows and went to battle. From the people living around the border, nine out of ten died. But just because he was lame, the old man and his son were both spared.

—from The Book of Lieh-tzu: A Classic of Tao, translated by Angus C. Graham

One-Minute Chapter Summary

Give yourself the gift of self-compassion. It gives you the space to question your self-critical assumptions. It gives you the ability to not berate yourself as hard for real or perceived mistakes.

Make a choice now:

- I choose to give myself the gift of self-compassion. I tell myself, "I am doing my very best with what I have in this moment, and that is all I can ask from myself."
- I choose to remain overly critical and judge every perceived imperfection as a mistake, possibly extrapolating that my life and my abilities are a mistake as well.

Head to http://bit.ly/youareenoughquiz to put in your answers, so that you can have a list of your affirmations and one-minute summaries to take with you after you finish reading the book.

CHAPTER 4. (YOU ARE WORTH OF THE GOLDEN TRIANGLE: SLEEP, EXERCISE, AND NOURISHMENT.

"If you begin to understand what you are without trying to change it, then what you are undergoes a transformation."
—Jiddu Krishnamurti

Do you ever notice that you get snippy or snappy when your blood sugar is low? Or that you are a different person without enough sleep, worse than Dr. Jekyll and Mr. Hyde? Or do you feel angry when you don't exercise?

If any of this touches a chord, then you're just like me.

I learned a new word from Facebook—"hangry." At first I thought someone had misspelt the country Hungary, or were perhaps hungry, but the word is actually a combination of "hungry" and "angry." Some people get very "hangry"—so much so that the chocolate peanutty nougat goodness of Snickers capitalized on it and made the negative feelings surrounding hunger a part of their branding in 2015. Notice the next time you've forgotten to eat—do you tend to get a bit short with yourself and others?

I am not going to expound that you need three meals a day with two snacks at 10 am and 3 pm, but I am going to say that you should listen to your body, and find doctors who listen to your body as well. As for me, my hangriness follows a predictable pattern. I eat breakfast at 7:30 am with my morning handful of pills. Then I start feeling hangry at around 10:30 am, so I satiate with a high quality fruit and nut trail mix. Between 1 and 2 pm, I finally head out for lunch, because I can't really focus after a big meal. Then I try to find something to eat again on my drive home at 5 pm. Dinner is around 6:30 or no later than 7:30 pm. But that's because I have kids and I try to have them asleep by 8:30 at night.

Sleep is another of those things you can't do without, despite what Silicon Valley, Corporate America, and the so-called "high achievers" say. The amount itself is important. You know how much sleep you need to function properly, and how much sleep you need to barely maneuver your vehicle through traffic, or get off on the right stop on the bus.

And if you don't know, you should learn as soon as possible. You have to live with yourself for the rest of your life, so it's paramount you get to know yourself, and sleep is a good place to start. If you feel particularly refreshed going to bed at 10:30 pm and waking up at 6:30 am, by all means, do it. You don't have to be a Tim Cook who sleeps six to seven hours a night. Sometimes you might need more sleep depending on what happened in the day. Sometimes you can get away with less sleep because you exercised enough during the day.

I'm not saying you should get seven hours of exercise followed by one hour of sleep. It doesn't work that way.

But exercise is important.

Getting the butt-off-chair is an important part of your life. If you have the patience and perseverance, it is important to get one hour of aerobic (you're sweating and visibly panting) exercise each day. I do feel better on the days I do exercise, even if I stay up until midnight and wake up at 6 am. On the other hand, if I don't get enough exercise—like when I broke my wrist—I am sluggish and snappy the following day and I need three more hours of sleep to even approximate how felt when I was exercising regularly.

That lasted for two months.

The hardest part is starting from a period of too much office time, too much kid time, too much not-enough-time-for-yourself. Try to hook a workout onto an existing habit that you have. Dr. B.J. Fogg, a well-known Stanford researcher and director of the Persuasive Tech Lab, says that you should take baby steps and change your environment in forming a successful habit. That means in the exercise example, you get an accountability partner—this changes your environment. He or she is responsible to check in with you every day to see if you exercised or not, at minimum. A really good accountability partner would go on to the gym with you.

The next part is connecting the association of going to the gym with an existing habit. For example, if you go to the coffee shop every morning, then commit to leaving the house an hour later or earlier to get your coffee, so that you still have time go to the gym. Over time—21 to 30 days, depending on the source—you will be able to go to the gym. The most important part is just taking action.

One-Minute Chapter Summary

Sleep, exercise, and food is incredibly important for your health. If you only choose two, you are like a stool with only two legs. You can't balance on that.

Make a choice now:

- I choose to make sure that I am getting enough sleep, nourishment, and exercise—even if it means pacing the stairs for 10 minutes a day—so that I will minimize being "hangry" or irritable.
- I choose to continue on my current path, even though I know that it is not sustainable in the long run, and may lead to a big wake-up call about my health down the road.

Head to http://bit.ly/youareenoughquiz to put in your answers, so that you can have a list of your affirmations and one-minute summaries to take with you after you finish reading the book.

CHAPTER 5. AS YOU ARE.

"Because one believes in oneself, one doesn't try to convince others. Because one is content with oneself, one doesn't need others' approval. Because one accepts oneself, the whole world accepts him or her."
—Lao Tzu

As I write these chapters further on in the book, it gets harder and harder to do. The words don't flow as well. It's because I haven't yet fully mastered accepting myself as I am. I know well enough that I am somewhere on the journey, but unsure of exactly where I am.

But I continue.

I think that self-acceptance is like a spectrum—there are some individuals that really are comfortable in their own skin and aren't afraid to be who they are. Then there's the rest of us, for whom, depending on the situation and the group of people around us, self-acceptance is a moving target.

But before you can accept yourself as you are, you need to know who you are.

Self-awareness is incredibly helpful. As you start detaching from society's expectations and your parents' exceptions, heck, even your spouse's expectations, you can start dusting all that sand off yourself, off your fossil, and start seeing it for what it really is.

Is that bone the forearm of a T-rex? Or is it Wyoming green fish from the Green River formation? Or is it a leaf? Or is something else entirely? You can make guesses about what you see, but until you delve further and dig deeper, and excavate all that dirt around the object, and try to minimize damage to that object, you will never know what it is that you found.

You may often go through your life without understanding the outline of who you actually are. You may be going on a journey, but you don't know why you started. Perhaps it's because all of your friends are marathon runners, so you decide that you should become one too. Who knows.

You do.

You need to look at yourself profoundly in the mirror. Let go of the parental expectations. Let go of societal expectations. And most importantly, let go of any expectations of yourself. You don't have to be that perfect mom who can socialize at a drop of the hat. You don't have to be the perfect engineer and get awards for your work. You don't have to be able to deal with all conflicts and get the preferred outcome the first time. You don't have to berate yourself every time you procrastinate talking with your boss because you're afraid of conflict.

Who would you be without any expectations of outcomes? Who would you be if you decided to opt out of your current identity? What if you went from a highly successful career woman with family to a stay-at-home mom—or the other way? Would you be able to put yourself in those shoes?

The great thing about accepting yourself as you are

today is, it also helps others understand and accept themselves. When other folks see you as being comfortable in your own skin, with your blemishes, and all of your so-called imperfections, then they can relax around you. They don't need to put on a mask to hide who or what they actually are, because you are presenting yourself as you are, nothing more, nothing less.

When you are okay with the fact that you have depression or diabetes or some other chronic condition that you'll probably have to deal with for the rest of your life, you lessen the tension internally. You stop fighting. You create peace for yourself.

One-Minute Chapter Summary

Create peace for yourself through first knowing who you are, then accepting who you are. The first step in knowing who you are is to drop everyone else's expectations of who you should be. The hardest expectations to let go of are your own hopes of who you should become.

Make a choice:

- I choose to let go of expectations of who I should be and what I should be doing with my life. I instead choose to accept who I am right now.
- I will continue to chase everyone's expectations and my own of what I should be doing. By choosing this path, I know that I am on the way to being unhappy and dissatisfied with myself.

Head to http://bit.ly/youareenoughquiz to put in your answers, so that you can have a list of your affirmations and one-minute summaries to take with you after you finish reading the book.

CHAPTER 6. TRUST YOURSELF.

"You can't connect the dots looking forward; you can only connect them looking backwards. So you have to trust that the dots will somehow connect in your future. You have to trust in something—your gut, destiny, life, karma, whatever. This approach has never let me down, and it has made all the difference in my life."
—Steve Jobs

Trust. When I think about all the connotations associated with that word, I have to laugh at its absurdity. I visualize cheesy team-building exercises, where one person closes her eyes, and then falls backward, presumably into the waiting arms of someone behind her. The trust game doesn't always work though. Especially if the person behind you is afraid of catching you as you fall. But implicit in the word "trust" is also "belief," which I learned the hard way when I was president of the Society of Women Engineers section in Houston.

This was my first time managing anybody face-to-face, and I had to see my volunteers every month, or more. My biggest failure in "leadership"—or it was more like, "Keep everyone on the ship!"—was in not trusting my team to come through for me, and vice versa.

I tried doing the treasurer's role and made a new Excel format for it. Bad idea. I helped a little too much at one event for the Vice President of Internal Affairs. I didn't help enough at another, where I needed to show up for an event with the Vice President of External Affairs. At one point, I got dehydrated so badly in between balancing work, volunteering, and the kids, that I had a fever of 101 degree Fahrenheit and my pulse was at about 120 beats per minute. I had to go to the urgent care clinic where the doctors gave me an IV drip of saline. Please refer to the section on "I am worthy."

I did recover from the dehydration. I did end up recovering from stretching myself too thin. I did eventually heal some of my health, to the best of my ability.

But I remember thinking after finishing my presidency and passing the gavel onto another engineer that, "Something has got to change."

My anxiety was getting so bad in Houston that any car that changed lane immediately in front of me was a cause for a panic attack. Going and talking to certain people in different disciplines and asking them questions was too much for me.

Something had to change.

But what really got me there was when my son got incredible heat rashes. They were particularly bad in the 100 percent humidity, coupled with a temperature of 95 degrees Fahrenheit or more. I remember when I was hosing him down with cool water in the shade, when he was thirteen months old, and that was still not enough to dampen the angry red welts dotting his body. I remember how utterly hopeless I felt. I handed the hose to my husband, powerless against Mother Nature and my son's biology.

But he still wanted to stay outside, despite the heat rash. On trips to Colorado during the holidays, he would want to stay outside in 10-degree weather. He had temper tantrums just so that he could be outside. His breath would create little clouds against the night sky, sometimes combining with mine when our breaths would be in unison.

I didn't fully realize how difficult change would be until I found the critical number and strength of supporters and friends who would point out the obvious to me. My son loved being outdoors, but by being in Houston, we were taking that away from him. My circle enabled me to really wake up and trust my own judgment and myself again.

In a way, I was similar to the chick in P.D. Eastman's *Are You My Mother?* In the book, the mother bird flies away to find food, leaving her egg in the nest. The egg hatches, and the chick asks a dog, a kitten, and a cow if anyone of them is his mother, but each in turn responds that he or she is not his mother. Finally, he meets up with the power shovel that returns the chick back to her nest just as her mother comes back to the nest. The vast majority of people out there are not there to give you support, but can provide some answers. What you really need are the power-shovel supporters, who give you the belief in yourself to literally thrust your way back home to honor your own inner voice.

This is how I woke up. Getting an executive coach from a good friend and finally being referred to the right psychiatrist probably helped. I didn't know that having the right people around me was going to make all the difference. Jim Rohn, a motivational speaker, says that you are the average of the five people you spend the most time with. Hopefully, these people are your power-shovel supporters.

For a while, or the six years I lived in Houston, I stopped trusting in myself and my own intuition. I wasn't happy, but I wasn't doing anything about it. Growing up next to the mountains in Colorado, and seeing the transparent streams of Clear Creek in college, I did not know what was wrong with me and Houston. The city was hot, flat, and humid. The rivers were large, muddy, somewhat polluted, and had water moccasins, a type of poisonous water snake.

For my children though, it became increasingly clear that Houston was not a good fit. My son had heat rashes whenever we let him outside during the summers. My daughter had pretty bad allergies and got sick at least once per month. It became apparent that Hand-Foot-and-Mouth disease was not a virus found in distant farmlands affecting cattle. She had that five separate times over the course of six months.

Still, we stayed in Houston and thought that everything would be all right, and that the corporation would take care of my husband and me, and move us up to Alaska as we had so politely asked.

The corporation was not going to send me and my husband to Alaska. There were going to be layoffs, and the price of oil was nose-diving—again. Luckily, I had my circle of mentors that personally believed in me, even if I didn't. These people are better than having a personal Board of Directors. They are your personal board of Angels on Earth. They shepherd you through the most difficult of times; they are your believers. You need your team. If you don't have a team, find them. I found my team by taking a chance and emailing somebody who I looked up to, who wrote a blog. She set me up with a good executive coach. You can find

both of them in the Acknowledgements section.
With a team on my side, and antidepressants that actually lifted me out of my drab mood and finally made me think clearly, I started believing in myself again.
Within six months, we had moved out of Houston to Alaska.
I found the same career in a different setting.
I took my kids skiing for the first time one year later. It was and still is one of my favorite winter sports.
I honored myself, and my family.
Trust yourself.

One-Minute Chapter Summary

Learn to trust yourself and your own judgment. Find your Circle of Mentors, or the people who never stop believing in you, even if you have stopped believing in yourself. Having your team in places enables you to make massive changes, despite the challenges ahead. They enable you to take small actions, one day at a time, to build your trust in yourself and in them.

Make a decision now:

- I resolve to trust myself and find trust in others by finding my Circle of Mentors, and naming one person in that circle now, and scheduling a half-hour session with that person via email.
- I cannot trust myself or others, and as a consequence, I am anxious, depressed, and scared. I don't know who will come through for me and I don't know who is on my power-shovel support team. I prefer to be blind to the trust and support that I can receive from the right group of people.

Head to http://bit.ly/youareenoughquiz to put in your answers, so that you can have a list of your affirmations and one-minute summaries to take with you after you finish reading the book.

CHAPTER 7. STOP THINKING AND START DOING.

The things to do are: the things that need doing, that you see need to be done, and that no one else seems to see need to be done."
—R.Buckminster Fuller

Somewhere in between ruminating about the past and getting depressed, and getting anxious about what the future holds, is the present moment. Being able to fully be in the present is a rare gift. I am so anxious right now, I am ready to jump out of my skin onto a football field and force myself to fit into a small safe place at the same time. But here I am, still writing.
Just do it.
It means stop thinking. It means to stop ruminating. What if you bought an app and it tracked how many times any particular negative thought came up? What would that counter say? One? Ten? One hundred? One thousand times you have thought this same thought, and fought it. At some point, you must act on your thoughts or let them go. There is a powerful quote about this:

Watch your thoughts, they become words;

watch your words, they become actions;
watch your actions, they become habits;
watch your habits, they become character;
watch your character, for it becomes your destiny.

— Frank Outlaw (Late President of the Bi-Lo Stores)

That's why taking action is so important. It took me six years to finally start writing this book. I did not say writing the rough draft. I mean it took me six years to finally extract my thoughts from my mind and overcome the fears and roadblocks that prevented me from even starting.

What made the change for me?

I finally got to know someone who had just released a book. Another gal who I knew halfway around the world, in Nigeria, was working on her second non-fiction book, and who is also a reservoir engineer—just like me. That was mind blowing in and of itself. I wanted to be a writer too. And she made me realize that it was possible to be a writer and an engineer, and that I just had to do it.

The random 200-word to 400-word blog posts I write may be completely trash, or close, when I share them on LinkedIn. But I get feedback. I start getting direct feedback on what people like. I ask them questions, like "What was your favorite part of that post?" or "What inspired you the most?"

But really, the hardest part is to just start doing it. Without doing it, you will never get any feedback. It will be stuck in a do-loop, forever swirling around in your mind like supercool helium— or for those of us who think in more concrete terms, it will be stuck in your mind like a cow chewing her cud over and over again, until it finally comes out the other end.

The real problem with letting your thoughts ruminate is that many of them never become action. Did you ever have a good idea for a book? When was the last time you actually sat down and wrote the outline? Did you ever have a good idea for your child's school webpage? Act on them!

By doing things, instead of thinking about the same things over and over again hundreds, or maybe even thousands of times, allows the outer world to give you feedback on your ideas. Good or bad, horrible or not, you have interacted with the world—and when you interact with the world, you learn.

Even if you aren't 100 percent successful on the first go, the pattern of acting on your thoughts and getting things done has a powerful multiplying effect on your life. It proves to you that even if you didn't get the most perfect, most prettiest product out the door, it means that you were able to act, and to make multiple decisions on what is important and what is not. It means that you are a person of action, and that you can slowly break out of the rumination of that single thought. It means that over time, you can become whoever you want to be. It means that you are trying to figure out what is better. It means you are becoming the best you.

Taking action makes you unique in this world. It gets you to the Dip, as Seth Godin writes about in his book with the same title. And with enough action and enough thinking about how to improve that action, you can get through The Dip to become the top of your field.

Maybe you are in the middle of The Dip right now. It's a less-then-optimal place to be making decisions, but it means that you are close to the breakthrough. Keep on taking action. Focus your time and energy on what really matters to you. Quit—which is also an action—everything else that takes away from that focus, which is how you achieve mastery. Keep on putting one foot in front of another, even if you don't want to.

That is the gift of action. It takes you places that you never thought to go.

And will you succeed?
Yes! You will, indeed!
(98 and 3/4 percent guaranteed.)

KID, YOU'LL MOVE MOUNTAINS!

So...
be your name Buxbaum or Bixby or Bray
or Mordecai Ali Van Allen O'Shea,
You're off to the Great Places!
Today is your day!
Your mountain is waiting.
So...get on your way!

— Dr. Seuss

One-Minute Chapter Summary

Taking a step, no matter how small, is the difference between success and failure. Over time, these steps snowball into a book, into blog posts, into a better relationship with your best friend or estranged mother.

Make a decision now:

- I commit to reaching out to somebody I admire who has done what I want to do, and scheduling a 15-minute session with him or her. I will take and do one task from that call.
- This goal is not a priority for me, so I am not reaching out.

Head to http://bit.ly/youareenoughquiz to put in your answers, so that you can have a list of your affirmations and one-minute summaries to take with you after you finish reading the book.

CHAPTER 8. PRACTICE PATIENCE.

"When I run after what I think I want, my days are a furnace of stress and anxiety; if I sit in my own place of patience, what I need flows to me, and without pain. From this, I understand that what I want also wants me, is looking for me, and attracting me. There is a great secret here for anyone who can grasp it."
—Rumi

Patience is the virtue I understand the least. Waiting is a foreign concept. I don't wait. I graduated high school a year early. I got into a magnet middle school in my school district. When I wanted to change elementary schools because I was correcting my second grade teacher in math, (my parents and) I made it happen. I always got what I wanted. I was, and am to this day, absolutely a spoiled brat.

So it was hard for me to go to my third choice school, despite getting accepted into both Wellesley and Smith for college. It was for financial reasons, and a real sense of practicality that my parents had, but I didn't at the time. I wanted to go study English at Smith but, in all reality, my parents kept on hinting at Colorado School of Mines. After all, I got a presidential scholarship to go to Mines.

Things do get better. Despite getting pregnant during my senior year at Mines, I still managed to graduate and secure an engineering job at an integrated oil and gas company. But then I had kids, and kids test patience the most of all.

So does depression. For me, it comes in waves of anger and overwhelms me, alternately pulsing in and out of my mind like the way the moon acts on the tides. So I start running away, and don't stop. Away from my kids within my mind, away from my job that felt so stressful. What all this boiled down to was that I wasn't patient enough with myself to just let events unfold and let myself be in the here and now. At one point, I was so impatient that I had to jump to the next to-do item on the list, without finishing the first thing. For example, I was unable to wait for water to boil for macaroni and cheese for the kids. So I went to vacuum, and forgot about the pot of boiling water entirely until one of them asked me again when lunch would be ready.

I fought the fact that I was a mom, until my daughter turned six and my son was about two years old. I existed most days in a paradoxical state, not really focused on where I was because I had some place better to be. At home, I wanted to be at the office and do some work in quiet and without the clash of my kids voices, their little cymbals smashing in on my perfectly orchestrated concert. Or more precisely, the office was home, and home was where I did the hardest work of my life. The kids were separate beings that I frustratingly couldn't control, and they emotionally drained me.

However, work was more or less under my control, or at least I knew what to expect. I could control my environment by putting on headphones. I couldn't do that with my kids.

Patience is letting events unfold within their own time. That is the beauty of it. It is about letting yourself be, not forcing yourself to fit a certain mold that you think you're ready for, but the universe has not yet agreed to. There are many obstacles in the way. I am not saying, "Don't fight through those obstacles," but rather, "Are the obstacles trying to tell you something?" That is the power of patience. It is sometimes about taking what you know already, and letting yourself bloom in whatever aspect it is that you desire.

If I follow patience, then I can do it—whatever it is. Sometimes—many times, since I am an engineer and mom—I hit a problem that I cannot figure out. These problems can be simple. For example, on a Saturday in February, I am going to a conference out of town. But my husband has to prepare a training for his field personnel by Monday. We have one au pair, who can only work 45 hours a week, has to have 36 hours off consecutively, and has a concert to go to on the Friday night. My husband and I talk about it and get frustrated. Here's where patience comes in. Instead of trying to solve the problem right now, take a moment away and do something else. We both cleaned the house and let the kids run around and find their own amusement, without causing any severe damage to themselves. After about an hour, we talked about it and things got better. Our au pair will watch the kids half a day on the Monday before, then I will watch the kids. And then our au pair can watch the kids half a day on Saturday, if necessary, so that my husband can prep for the training

if he has to.
Patience is also crucial for making life decisions. Sometimes, you hit a period of life where many opportunities come at you, and you don't know what to say. Yes, or no? Should you overburden yourself with the obligations that these opportunities become? Practice some patience. Wanting to answer at the time the speaker asks for it is impractical and gives you imperfect expectations. Sleep on it for a night. Wait and see what happens. Sometimes, whoever is asking may find someone else to do the task if you just wait to give a response.
But what if you don't have enough opportunities? Here too, practice patience. What is it that you are lacking, in terms of skills, thinking, or mindset? Have you helped out someone else? Often, you need to help someone else first achieve their goals before you can achieve your own. Practice patience here too, while doing consistent work towards your goals to achieve those opportunities.
I've found that in patience, there is immense peace. You are a lion, fully aware, fully awake, but holding yourself calmly, waiting patiently for prey. There is peace in the waiting. There is peace in rejoicing in the now, in not having the opportunity that you covet so badly right now. Why? When you have the patience to enjoy this moment, instead of ruminating somewhere in the past or having anxiety about the future, then you can fully be here. Being here awakens you to the possibilities and opportunities that this moment provides, and because you are aware, the opportunities present themselves. Like a lion hiding in wait, the prey appears, and you are able to see it because you are not clouded by your thoughts of yesterday or tomorrow; then you pounce, and you are ready for a warm meal.

Patience provides a certain level of peace.
Practice patience.
Practice awareness in this moment.

One-Minute Chapter Summary

Patience is the virtue least understood. If you can find it and let events simply unfold as they are, there is minimal fighting over the outcome of that event. When you are patient with yourself, you become more aware of the present, and thus of any opportunities that may present themselves. Impatience puts the blinders on in many situations, which increases the chance for blunders.

Make a decision now:

- The next time I am doing something I find really frustrating—like having my five-year-old read to me, I will take a moment and take a breath in. I will tell myself that it's all right to have more patience towards my child and myself. She will learn to read eventually, and I need to give her some patience to learn how to read in kindergarten.
- I don't understand why being patient is useful to me.

Head to http://bit.ly/youareenoughquiz to put in your answers, so that you can have a list of your affirmations and one-minute summaries to take with you after you finish reading the book.

EPILOGUE

I have realized; it is during the times I am far outside my element that I experience myself the most. That I see and feel who I really am, the most! I think that's what a comet is like, you see, a comet is born in the outer realms of the universe! But it's only when it ventures too close to our sun or to other stars that it releases the blazing "tail" behind it and shoots brazen through the heavens! And meteors become sucked into our atmosphere before they burst like firecrackers and realize that they're shooting stars! That's why I enjoy taking myself out of my own element, my own comfort zone, and hurling myself out into the unknown. Because it's during those scary moments, those unsure steps taken, that I am able to see that I'm like a comet hitting a new atmosphere: suddenly I illuminate magnificently and fire dusts begin to fall off of me! I discover a smile I didn't know I had, I uncover a feeling that I didn't know existed in me... I see myself. I'm a shooting star. A meteor shower. But I'm not going to die out. I guess I'm more like a comet then. I'm just going to keep on coming back.

—C. JoyBell C.

Here I am, sitting on my computer at 12:30 am on a Saturday night, probably contradicting everything I wrote about on sleep—but I feel satisfied. Through writing this book, I'm letting go of a lot of the old angers and hurts and attempting to rewire my brain's thought habits. I am still trying to rewire my if-then thought networks, and I'm taming my amygdala, or fight-flight-freeze portion of my brain that overrides higher critical thinking in the cortex.

It all starts with the belief that you are worth it. I can't prove it to you—there is no geometric proof for that. I just know. But if you are reading this book right now, and you've gotten all the way to the end, you are worth it, my friend. Even if you stopped reading in the middle of the book, you are worth it. Even if you never picked up this book in your life, you're worth it.

Believe that you are worth it when you are ruminating about how you are not good enough, about how you are overwhelmed by life's small, insignificant events—being late to a class, when your child gets sick with a fever for the first time, when you slide on ice and break your wrist.

It's okay. You will learn and grow and eventually move out of this phase of your life and find a new phase.

You are worth it.

Believe it.

You are worth it.

THE MIRROR IN THE CORNER

For a long time, I was deeply afraid of my past. And sometimes, I still am.

I was incredibly sensitive to my mom's criticism. She yelled at me on a regular basis. Why wasn't I better? What was wrong with me? Why couldn't I have perfect Chinese calligraphy? I was the only child. She gave up a lot for me, and I perceived at times, she deeply resented me.

Those childhood memories still drive a lot of my reactions.

My mother's reactions became my reactions. Her criticality became mine. I became judgmental of everyone I met, and especially those I met on the road. I would imagine stories about them, that I was better than them, and they were in my way, impeding my progress. I felt incredibly shamed and guilty that that's how I felt about my fellow human beings.

I would criticize myself so much, I would become anxious when I didn't arrive at a place I thought I should already have arrived at. Not only when I was late in the car, but also in my career, which is where I derived a lot of my self-worth.

But recently, I've started to wake up. I became tired of the waves of anxiety and depression. To date, I have spent thousands on therapy, and many hours meditating and doing yoga, but only now have started to wake up.

What happened?

I looked into the hardest mirror: the one our mother holds up for us.

My mom came to help out when my eight-month old son was not sleeping through the night in January. I couldn't handle the lack of sleep, and needed to perform at my job, and was overwhelmed with negative self-talk, and was away from the house from 6:30 am to 7 pm and—well there are a lot of "ands." Needless to say, I thought that having my mom over for about eight weeks would be enough to bridge the gap and get me through the tough spot.

In the end, she lasted six weeks until she boarded an airplane and went back home in a different state.

During this time, I saw things transpire in my four-year-old daughter that hit close to home. Actually, I mean at home.

My daughter started showing signs of depression—crying, and a lot more crying than usual. She felt abandoned—my mom was taking care of my son, and my husband and I were too tired to do too much with her after we came home from work. She wet her pants three times a week.

But during the weekends, my mom would constantly nag my daughter to do her homework. She consistently criticized my husband and I about why we weren't reading more to her. She criticized my husband and I for letting her watch too many movies during the weekend. My mom thought that she could raise my child better than me. It was never enough for my mom. But she didn't propose any solutions.

The mirror was being held up, and it was eerily similar.

I remember when my mom was comparing my Chinese character handwriting with another boy's when I was in first grade, who was one year younger than me. His characters were so much squarer, so much more symmetrical and just so much more perfect than mine. The worst thing was that she taught the Chinese language class. There were only three students in the class, including the miniature Chinese-character-writing genius child and myself. I drowned my inadequacies and imperfections in the KFC mashed potato and gravy at the end of each class. I did not want my daughter to suffer the same fate that I had.

She did not, and has not. We are teaching her to embrace and honor who she is. No matter what, she is enough.

THANK YOU

Before you go, I'd like to say "thank you" for purchasing the manifesto.

I know you could have picked from dozens of books on women's self-help. But you took a chance with my manifesto. So a big thanks for downloading this book and reading all the way to the end. If you like what you've read, I need your help.

Please take a moment and leave a review of my book on Amazon by heading to this address: http://youareenough.co.

This feedback will help me continue to write the kind of Kindle books that help you get results.

Cheers!

GRATITUDE

I would like to thank the teams of people I've encountered throughout my life; these teams have kept me glued together and alive. They've taken me from the edge; they've reminded me who I am when I judge myself in the worst ways possible. They've tapped me on the shoulder when I was ready to jump from the top of the north parking garage. These are the people who found ways into my life at critical turning points, when I wasn't ready, or didn't think I was ready, to grow.

This section, I assume, will grow with each book. I want to memorialize each person, so that they have a gift of sorts to carry them forward, and to know that they made a difference in at least one person's life in their storied path. They made a difference when our paths crossed, ran parallel, and then their path disappeared while I continued on mine.

Miss White and Miss McAfoos—you both taught at Mission Viejo Elementary. Thank you for teaching me about the beauty of poetry and of listening closely to hear the real message being transmitted. Thank you for exposing me to different cultures and making me remember that we are were all refugees at one point.

Mrs. Anderson—you taught me in your Humanities class at Challenge School. You taught me about project management, and how life is ultimately a mystery to be teased apart. You taught me that I could write, and to never stop believing in myself.

Mrs. Bartholomew—you taught me so much about chemistry and to keep on preserving in the quest for knowledge. I still remember the clementines you gave us during Science Bowl and AP Chemistry study sessions at your house.

Dr. Ramona Graves —you kept believing in me and kept me in Petroleum Engineering after I failed my first structural geology test. You recommended playdough to solve my problems and to pass structural geology. Playdough is useful for building all sorts of structures, and is a good source of profound stress relief.

Dr. Jennifer Miskimins, P.E.—you are just a constant in the Mines petroleum engineering department that I continue to turn to for advice and guidance at key inflection points in my life.

Jill Cooper—an amazing boss who taught me that whether in the public or private sector, you have to treat people with humanity, and to be gentle with them.

Katie Mehnert, Sonya Ware, Stephanie Frey, and Dr. Claudia Orengo—I can write a book about how you four put my life back together in Houston and enabled our move to Anchorage during an oilfield downturn.

Jill Tietjen, P.E.—my Society of Women Engineers believer and constant companion, mentor, friend, and constant source of belief and faith. Sometimes I suspect that she is a more seasoned version of myself.

Jennifer Braganza—my book coach and someone who challenges my thinking around my book and my priorities. You kept me on track to deliver—my book, my life, and my important people.

My parents, my family, my kids, my husband—one day,

when I have healed from the trauma of raising a family, having a full-time career, volunteering, and writing a book, then I can fully dedicate a volume (or two!) to the ever changing, dynamic madness that is a product of the environment, genetics, and pure genius.

Isabel Pansegrau—for better or worse, you saw the worst of me and still had to live with us for a year as our au pair. Thanks for taking care of my kids so I could focus on my day job.

ABOUT THE AUTHOR

Islin Munisteri is an engineer by day, writer by night, and keeps her depression at bay by writing and volunteering. She lives in Alaska, in the United States, with her husband, two kids, and 15 (plus or minus five) chickens, and her dog named Suki.

You can find her on www.islinmunisteri.com, islinmunisteri@me.com, Twitter (@munisteri), LinkedIn, and Facebook. You can also find her 501(c)3 nonprofit on Facebook if you search for Creating Potential (and make sure it's the one based in the United States).

69690418R00043

Made in the USA
Middletown, DE
08 April 2018